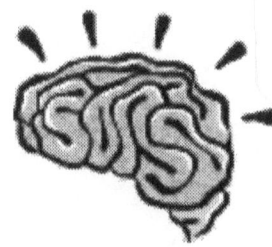

# BrainReady

# BrainChallenge 2

Helping you fight mental aging - the easy
& convenient way

## Jim Balabuszko-Reay
## and Paul Sebastien

Written by Jim Balabuszko-Reay
and Paul Sebastien

www.brainready.com
info@brainready.com

Published by Lulu.com
www.lulu.com

ISBN: 978-1-4303-2956-5

# Welcome!
## Ready for More Challenges?

The brain is a wonderful thing. Just think where you'd be without one! But starting from around age 25, our brains begin to deteriorate, with each passing year: memory, speed, recall, overall brainpower. Fortunately, recent research has shown that there's actually something you can do about that: brain exercises!

Exercise is not just for bodies anymore. Studies have shown that doing creative, spatial and memory-challenging exercises can actually help prevent brain deterioration and even help recover lost function. That's right: just like your physical body, it's "Use it or Lose it".

Interestingly, studies have also shown that traditional brain teasers and tough puzzles are not as beneficial to brain health as repeated, simpler exercises that work *several* areas of the brain. Just like doing a comprehensive physical cross-training workout is better for your overall health than, say, only doing bench presses.

With this in mind, we have created this SECOND SET of BrainChallenge exercises, intended to help you cross train your brain while making it FUN, and easy. You won't find any trivia here, nor any math, logic, or any other puzzles. This book is dedicated to exercising your memory and creativity. The only think you'll need is a pencil and your brain.

Here's what you'll find in the pages that follow...

### Recall:

In these exercises, you're challenged to recall events from long ago or earlier today, from major life events to everyday details. Variations include answering short questions, writing out longer stories, or drawing objects from memory. New in this edition are musical recall challenges, as well as exercises to challenge your observation throughout the day.

The ultimate goal is not just to remember these items, but to *unclog and reawaken* your memory capacity, which can help your past, present and future memory power!

### Creative

Drawing, creative writing, poetry – it's all here to help exercise your brain. Don't worry if you don't feel like an "artist" - the important thing is that you just *try* each one. We've expanded the number of creative challenges this round, including new "It's a Theory" exercises. You'll find all of these challenges deliver a truly comprehensive workout for your brain.

### Switch-Up

Some exercises ask that you do it twice: from writing from two points of view, drawing multiple sides of an object, to drawing and writing with both hands. These force you to use different areas of your brain and really fire those synapses in new ways!

We hope you enjoy these exercises, and that doing them helps you truly FEEL your brain re-awakening. But most importantly, we hope that you HAVE FUN cross-training your brain!

For more information on Brain Health, be sure to visit
www.brainready.com

## Now, on to the BrainChallenge!

## BrainChallenge™ - Draw From Memory

Category: Recall          Difficulty: Medium

## Draw a piece of art from your home

Drawing from Memory exercises your critical Spatial and Memory brain areas as well as brain-motor skills. It can be especially hard to remember details of something you look at every single day!

Category: Recall          Difficulty: Easy

## What were you doing yesterday at 10 am?

_____

_____

_____

_____

## What were you doing at 3:30pm Yesterday?

_____

_____

_____

_____

It can be surprising how short-term details can be _harder_ to recall than older, but larger, life events.  Spend a few moments and really try to remember the details...

## BrainChallenge™ - It's a Theory

Category: Creative          Difficulty: Medium

# Where does art come from?

_____

_____

_____

_____

_____

_____

_____

_____

_____

The key with "It's a Theory" is to come up with a creative, possibly plausible, possibly funny explanation to the question posed. Have fun and use your imagination!

## BrainChallenge™ - Haiku

Category: Creative          Difficulty: Easy

## Write a Haiku about the thaw in Spring

_____

_____

_____

## Now, write a Haiku about budding leaves

_____

_____

_____

### HOW TO HAIKU:

Haiku is a Japanese Poetry Form:
The first line is 5 syllables
The second line is 7 syllables
The third is 5
It need not rhyme!

Writing in haiku forces you to think differently about language, to express yourself in a new way, which is an *excellent* creative, translative exercise for your brain!

| Category: Recall | Difficulty: Medium |

# Who were your Elementary School Teachers?

First Year: _____

Second Year: _____

Third Year: _____

Fourth Year: _____

Fifth Year: _____

See what other details you can recall about these teachers...
their first names, the color of their hair, the sound of their
voices, classes you may have enjoyed (or not)

Spending time on these details is excellent brain exercise!

## BrainChallenge™ - Left Hand Drawing

**Category:  Switch-Up**          **Difficulty:  Medium**

## Draw a Flower with your LEFT HAND

Drawing the same object with the right and left hand illustrates
how hand preference is "hard wired" into our brains....

## BrainChallenge™ - Right Hand Drawing

**Category: Switch-Up**    **Difficulty: Medium**

## Draw a Flower with your RIGHT HAND

... and by forcing your non-dominant hand to try to do the same task as your dominant one, you are forcing your brain into a tough, comprehensive "adaptation" workout!

**Category:  Recall**          **Difficulty:  Hard**

Hum a theme from a classical symphony.

(Let it pop into your head!)

Who was the Composer?

_____

What is the name of the piece?

_____

When was the piece written (roughly)?

_____

The melody of a piece of music will stick in your mind far easier than any of the details about the piece.  Really try to remember the details about this piece.  Now that you've got the info, you can go find that CD and enjoy it in full!

| Category: Creative | Difficulty: Medium |

## List seven things you Love

_____

_____

_____

_____

_____

_____

_____

**Self-examination makes for very good mental exercise.
Limiting to just seven can be a challenge!**

**Category:  Recall**          **Difficulty:  Hard**

## Write in as many languages as you can:
## Who are you?

_____

_____

_____

_____

_____

_____

_____

_____

_____

Learning and using languages is great brain exercise.

If you don't know any other languages, why not think of
several ways to say it in your own language?

## BrainChallenge℠ - Draw from Memory

**Category: Recall**          **Difficulty: Medium**

## Draw the light over your dining room table

Drawing from Memory exercises hand-eye coordination, and pushes you to recall fine detail as well as general size and shape relationships.

Category:  Switch-Up          Difficulty:  Medium

## Why were the Roman Gods better than the Greek Gods?

_____

_____

_____

_____

_____

_____

_____

_____

_____

_____

In point counterpoint, try to make a good case for BOTH SIDES of the argument.  It forces you to examine your assumptions and bias...

Category: Switch-Up        Difficulty: Medium

## Why were the Greek Gods better than the Roman Gods?

_____

_____

_____

_____

_____

_____

_____

_____

_____

_____

By giving a small area to write, your brain is forced to channel creativity and information prioritization!

## Your mission today:

### Count all of the RED CARS you see

### Bonus Mission:

### How many DELIVERY VANS did you see?

Keep your eyes open for the next 24 hours and try to keep this count in your head. Actively keeping watch for things in your environment keeps your brain active throughout the day!

Category: Creative          Difficulty: Medium

## Why does the wind blow?

_____

_____

_____

_____

_____

_____

_____

_____

_____

The key with "It's a Theory" is to come up with a creative, possibly plausible, possibly funny explanation to the question posed. Have fun and use your imagination!

Category: Creative          Difficulty:  Medium

## Write exactly 25 words about:
## Your Favorite Film

_____

_____

_____

_____

_____

_____

_____

_____

_____

_____

Expressing yourself within a fixed set of rules can force you to explore different words and sentence structures, which is good brain exercise.

Category: Recall          Difficulty: Hard

## How many beverages have you drunk in the past 24 hours?

_____

_____

## Name them!

_____

_____

_____

_____

_____

_____

It can be surprising how short term details can be harder to recall than larger life events.  Spend a few moments and really try to remember these details.

## BrainChallenge™ - Mirror Draw

Category: Switch-Up          Difficulty: Medium

**Draw the glass door to your detective agency, with your name on the glass**

Have fun with this - Recall your favorite film noir scene.

**Category:** Switch-Up          **Difficulty:** Medium

## Draw that glass door, viewed from INSIDE

The name on the door should be reversed... right?

Category: Recall          Difficulty: Medium

## What Musical Instruments have you learned how to play?

_____

_____

_____

_____

## Which ones can you still play?

_____

_____

Don't forget to include instruments you may have played in early grade-school orchestras or bands.

Playing music is fantastic exercise for your brain and your spirit.  Perhaps you should pick up that old instrument and get to know it again!

## BrainChallenge™ - Haiku

| Category: Creative | Difficulty: Medium |
| --- | --- |

### Write a Haiku about anything...
### and use the word "Gleam"

_____

_____

_____

### Now, write a Haiku about the North Star:

_____

_____

_____

### HOW TO:

Haiku is a Japanese Poetry Form:
The first line is 5 syllables
The second line is 7 syllables
The third is 5
It need not rhyme!

Writing in verse or haiku forces you to think differently about language, to express yourself in a new way, which is excellent exercise for your brain!

Category: Creative          Difficulty: Medium

## List seven things you Dislike

_____

_____

_____

_____

_____

_____

_____

Self-examination makes for very good mental exercise.
Limiting to just seven can be a challenge!

Category:  Recall          Difficulty:  Medium

## Hum a Movie Theme.

## (Let it pop into your head!)

## What was the movie?

_____

## Who was the star of this film?

_____

## When did this movie come out?

_____

The melody of a piece of music will stick in your mind far easier than any of the details about the piece.  Try to remember it all the way through.

**Category: Creative**          **Difficulty: Easy**

## Draw a Zeppelin

Drawing from Memory exercises hand-eye coordination, and
pushes you to recall fine detail as well as general size and
shape relationships.

## BrainChallenge™ - It's a Theory

Category: Creative          Difficulty: Medium

# Why aren't we flung into space as the Earth spins?

_____

_____

_____

_____

_____

_____

_____

_____

_____

The key with "It's a Theory" is to come up with a creative, possibly plausible, possibly funny explanation to the question posed. Have fun and use your imagination!

## BrainChallenge™ - Language

**Category: Recall**          **Difficulty: Hard**

## Write in as many languages as you can:
## Where am I?

---

---

---

---

---

---

---

---

---

Learning and using languages is great brain exercise.

If you don't know any other languages, why not think of as many ways to say it in your own language?

Category:  Creative          Difficulty:  Medium

## Write exactly 25 words about:
## Your Best Teacher

_____

_____

_____

_____

_____

_____

_____

_____

_____

Expressing yourself within a fixed set of rules can force you to explore different words and sentence structures, which is good brain exercise.

Category: Switch-Up          Difficulty: Medium

# Why would having three arms be better than having only two arms?

_____

_____

_____

_____

_____

_____

_____

_____

_____

_____

In point counterpoint, try to make a good case for BOTH SIDES
of the argument.  It forces you to examine your assumptions
and bias...

## Why would having two arms be better than having three arms?

_____

_____

_____

_____

_____

_____

_____

_____

_____

_____

By giving a small area to write, we are encouraging economy
in writing and creative wording.

## BrainChallenge™ - Haiku

**Category:  Creative**          **Difficulty:  Easy**

### Write a Haiku about Time

_____

_____

_____

### Now, write a Haiku about Thyme

_____

_____

_____

---

### HOW TO HAIKU:

Haiku is a Japanese Poetry Form:
The first line is 5 syllables
The second line is 7 syllables
The third is 5
It need not rhyme!

---

Writing in verse or haiku forces you to think differently about language, to express yourself in a new way, which is excellent exercise for your brain!

**Category: Recall          Difficulty: Medium**

# What were the FIRST words you said to another person today?

_____

_____

_____

_____

# What did they say in return?

_____

_____

_____

_____

Spend a few moments and really try to remember these details.
Recall of the most innocuous events in the day can be a great
brain workout.

## BrainChallenge™ - Left Hand Drawing

**Category: Switch-Up**     **Difficulty: Medium**

## Draw a Sun, Moon, and Star
## with your LEFT HAND

Drawing the same objects with the right and left hand shows
how hand preference is "hard wired" into our brains....

## BrainChallenge™ - Right Hand Drawing

**Category: Switch-Up**     **Difficulty: Medium**

## Draw a Sun, Moon and Star
## with your RIGHT HAND

... by forcing your non-dominant hand to try to do the same task as your dominant one, you are actually working some seldom used areas of your brain

Category: Recall                    Difficulty: Medium

## What was your first Car?

_____

## Where did you get it?

_____

## What happened to it?

_____

## What color was the exterior?  Interior?

_____

You may find that as you do other exercises, these answers
come to you.  That's your brain getting more fit!

**Category:  Creative**          **Difficulty:  Easy**

## Write about 7 things you:
## Admire

_____

_____

_____

_____

_____

_____

_____

Examining your beliefs and assumptions makes for very good
mental exercise.  Limiting to just seven can be a challenge!

**Category: Creative**          **Difficulty: Hard**

## Write 25 words about
## Something you'll never do again

_____

_____

_____

_____

_____

_____

_____

_____

_____

Let your imagination run wild... within 25 words of course!
Working creatively within constraints is a great workout.

**Category: Recall**          **Difficulty: Medium**

## Draw the label from your favorite coffee or tea package

Drawing from Memory exercises hand-eye coordination, and pushes you to recall fine detail.  No fair peeking at the package!

## BrainChallenge℠ - Mission: Observation

| Category: Recall | Difficulty: Medium |
| --- | --- |

### Your mission today:

Look for a person arguing on a cellphone.

### How many did you find?

### Bonus Mission:

How many people did you see LAUGHING
on a cellphone?

Keep your eyes open for the next 24 hours and try to keep this
count in your head. Actively keeping watch for things in your
environment keeps your brain active throughout the day!

**Category: Recall**          **Difficulty: Hard**

## Write in as many languages as you can:
## What time is it?

_____

_____

_____

_____

_____

_____

_____

_____

Learning and using languages is great brain exercise.

If you don't know any other languages, why not think of as many ways to say it in your own language?

| Category: Switch Up | Difficulty: Medium |
|---|---|

## Write with your LEFT Hand:

### The Title of your Favorite Book, along with the Author and lead character's name

_____

_____

_____

Writing with the right and left hand shows some unique ways in which hand preference is "hard wired" into our brains....

**Category:** Switch Up      **Difficulty:** Medium

## Write with your RIGHT Hand:

## The Title of your Favorite Book, along with the Author and lead character's name

_____

_____

_____

It's amazing how the same words and letters can look so different when produced by your non-dominant hand, isn't it?

Category: Recall          Difficulty: Medium

## Draw an Umbrella

Try to remember key details - how the ribs curve, how it looks
underneath.  Or you can draw it closed!

Category: Creative          Difficulty:  Medium

## Write exactly 25 words about:
## A Close Call

_____

_____

_____

_____

_____

_____

_____

_____

_____

_____

Expressing yourself within a fixed set of rules can force you to explore different words and sentence structures, which is good brain exercise.

**Category:** Switch-Up          **Difficulty:** Medium

## Why are Lungs better than Gills?

_____

_____

_____

_____

_____

_____

_____

_____

_____

_____

Try to make a good case for BOTH SIDES of the argument. It forces you to examine your assumptions and bias...

Category: Switch-Up          Difficulty: Medium

## Why are Gills better than Lungs?

_____

_____

_____

_____

_____

_____

_____

_____

_____

This time, it's a completely non-controversial topic, and you'll be challenged to make a case for either side... but still you must try!

| Category: Creative | Difficulty: Medium |
|---|---|

## Write a Haiku about Trains

_____

_____

_____

## Now, write a Haiku using the following two words: "Station" and "Pass"

_____

_____

_____

### HOW TO HAIKU:

Haiku is a Japanese Poetry Form:
The first line is 5 syllables
The second line is 7 syllables
The third is 5

Writing in verse or haiku forces you to think differently about language, to express yourself in a new way, which is excellent exercise for your brain!

## BrainChallenge™ - Seven Things

**Category:** Creative          **Difficulty:** Medium

# List seven things you are an Expert in

_____

_____

_____

_____

_____

_____

_____

Self-examination makes for very good mental exercise.
Limiting to just seven can be a challenge!

## BrainChallenge™ - Left Hand Drawing

Category: Switch-Up          Difficulty: Medium

## Draw a Triangle, Square, Pentagon, and Hexagon with your LEFT HAND

Drawing the same objects with the right and left hand shows
how hand preference is "hard wired" into our brains....

**Category: Switch-Up**     **Difficulty: Medium**

## Draw a Triangle, Square, Pentagon, and Hexagon with your LEFT HAND

... and by using your non-dominant hand, you are actually working some seldom used areas of your brain

Category: Recall          Difficulty: Medium

In your home:

How many doors lead to the outside?

_____

How many water faucets are there?

_____

How many radios are in your home?

_____

Recalling minute details of your everyday environment forces your brain to access some memories that may be elided over in everyday life, and may help activate other memory recall as well!

## What was the very FIRST image you saw on television last time you turned it on?

_____

_____

_____

## What was the very FIRST thing you heard on the radio last time you turned it on?

_____

_____

_____

Try to remember exactly what you saw or heard when your hand hit that power button... perhaps it was an ad?

Category: Creative          Difficulty: Medium

## Where do kittens come from?

_____

_____

_____

_____

_____

_____

_____

_____

_____

_____

The key with "It's a Theory" is to come up with a creative, possibly plausible, possibly funny explanation to the question posed. Have fun and use your imagination!

## Hum an Advertising Jingle.

### (Let it pop into your head!)

### What was the product?

_____

### What show would the ad appear during?

_____

### When was this ad on the air?

_____

The melody of a piece of music will stick in your mind far easier
than any of the details about the piece. Really try to
remember the details about this piece.
They sure don't write jingles like they used to.

57

**Category: Creative**          **Difficulty: Medium**

## Write 25 words about
## Someone you Miss

_____

_____

_____

_____

_____

_____

_____

_____

_____

_____

This one may be hard to keep to 25 words, but rise to the challenge.  Then spend some time reflecting further on you memory.

**Category: Creative**     **Difficulty: Medium**

## Draw a lightning bolt striking a tree

Be as detailed as you can - show the clouds and surrounding landscape as you can.

## BrainChallenge™ - Left Hand Writing

| Category:  Switch Up | Difficulty:  Hard |
|---|---|

### Write your MAILING ADDRESS
### with your LEFT Hand:
### Twice please:

_____

_____

_____

_____

Writing with the right and left hand shows some unique ways in
which hand preference is "hard wired" into our brains, and
your signature is one of the hardest to switch hands on.

## Write your MAILING ADDRESS
## with your RIGHT Hand:
## Twice please:

———————————————————————

———————————————————————

———————————————————————

———————————————————————

It's amazing how something as common as your address looks quite different when produced by your non-dominant hand.

Category: Creative          Difficulty: Medium

## Write a Haiku about your Toes

_____

_____

_____

## Now, write a Haiku about using the words "Market" and "Home"

_____

_____

_____

### HOW TO HAIKU:

Haiku is a Japanese Poetry Form:
The first line is 5 syllables
The second line is 7 syllables
The third is 5

Writing in verse or haiku forces you to think differently about language, to express yourself in a new way, which is excellent exercise for your brain!

## BrainChallenge™ - Creative Drawing

| Category: Creative | Difficulty: Easy |
|---|---|

## Draw a man with a mustache

As you draw, try to imagine this person's story - who is he?
What era is he from?

## Name ALL of the ingredients on your dinner plate last night.

_____

_____

_____

_____

## How about your most recent meal?

_____

_____

_____

_____

Take a guess on the ingredients of a sauce or puree. It's interesting that we often don't think about the constituent parts of our meals... it's good to pay attention!

## BrainChallenge™ - It's a Theory

Category: Creative          Difficulty: Medium

## How do telephones work?

_____

_____

_____

_____

_____

_____

_____

_____

_____

The key with "It's a Theory" is to come up with a creative,
possibly plausible, possibly funny explanation to the question
posed. Have fun and use your imagination!

**Category: Recall**         **Difficulty: Hard**

## Write in as many languages as you can:
## Do you speak English?

_____

_____

_____

_____

_____

_____

_____

_____

Learning and using languages is great brain exercise.

If you don't know any other languages, why not think of as many ways to say it in your own language?

**Category: Creative**  **Difficulty: Medium**

## Write 25 words about Birds

_____

_____

_____

_____

_____

_____

_____

_____

_____

Working creatively within constraints is excellent brain exercise.
Having goals in life is excellent all-around.

## BrainChallenge™ - Topsy Drawing

**Category:  Switch-Up**      **Difficulty:  Medium**

## Draw the Mona Lisa from Memory

Drawing from Memory exercises hand-eye coordination, and
pushes you to recall fine detail.

| Category: Switch-Up | Difficulty: HARD |
| --- | --- |

## Draw the Mona Lisa UPSIDE DOWN

Don't turn the book upside down - try to draw it upside down -
using your previous page drawing as a guide.
NOT EASY, is it?

## BrainChallenge™ - Music Memory

Category: Recall          Difficulty: Hard

Hum a theme from a TV Show.

(Let it pop into your head!)

What was the show?

_____

Who was the star of the show?

_____

What year did the show air?

_____

The melody of a piece of music will stick in your mind far easier
than any of the details about the piece.  Now, as you
remember the song, try to visualize the show's opening credits
to accompany it.

## BrainChallenge™ - Haiku

| Category: Creative | Difficulty: Medium |
|---|---|

### Write a Haiku about a Child

_____

_____

_____

### Now, write a Haiku about the Spirit of Youth

_____

_____

_____

### HOW TO HAIKU:

Haiku is a Japanese Poetry Form:
The first line is 5 syllables
The second line is 7 syllables
The third is 5
It need not rhyme!

Writing in verse or haiku forces you to think differently about language, which is excellent exercise for your brain!

Category: Switch-Up          Difficulty: Medium

## Why is flying a better superpower than invisibility?

_____

_____

_____

_____

_____

_____

_____

_____

_____

_____

Try to make a good case for BOTH SIDES of the argument. It forces you to examine your assumptions and bias...

## Why is invisibility a better superpower than flying?

_____

_____

_____

_____

_____

_____

_____

_____

_____

In this case, you'll definitely want to consider all of the pros and cons of each... this is important stuff!

## BrainChallenge™ - Seven Things

**Category: Creative**          **Difficulty: Medium**

## List seven things you don't understand

_____

_____

_____

_____

_____

_____

_____

Self-examination makes for very good mental exercise.
Limiting to just seven can be a challenge!

Category: Recall          Difficulty: Medium

## Draw the label of your favorite candy bar

Drawing from Memory pushes you to recall fine detail on common objects you may not be paying close attention to. No fair looking at the wrapper!

**Category: Creative**          **Difficulty: Medium**

## Why do oceans have tides?

_____

_____

_____

_____

_____

_____

_____

_____

_____

The key with "It's a Theory" is to come up with a creative, possibly plausible, possibly funny explanation to the question posed. Have fun and use your imagination!

Category: Recall          Difficulty: Medium

## Who was your first Best Friend?

_____

## How did you meet?

_____

_____

_____

## Are you still friends, or did you have a falling out?

_____

Don't worry if you can't recall every detail right away. You may find that as you do other unrelated exercises, these memories will come to you. That's your brain unclogging those cobwebs!

**Category: Switch Up**     **Difficulty: Medium**

## Write with your LEFT Hand:

## The Title of your Favorite TV Show, along with the Star and Network

_____

_____

_____

Writing with the right and left hand shows some unique ways in which hand preference is "hard wired" into our brains....

Category:  Switch Up          Difficulty:  Medium

## Write with your RIGHT Hand:

## The Title of your Favorite TV Show, along with the Star and Network

_____

_____

_____

It's amazing how the same words and letters can look so
different when produced by your non-dominant hand, isn't it?

Category: Creative          Difficulty: Easy

## Draw a Prehistoric Fish
## (that lives DEEP in the sea)

Have fun with this one!

## BrainChallenge™ - Mission: Observation

Category: Recall          Difficulty: Medium

Your mission today:

Watch the skies:  How many airplanes do
you see in the air?

Bonus Mission:

How about other flying machines
(helicopters, zeppelins, jetpacks?)

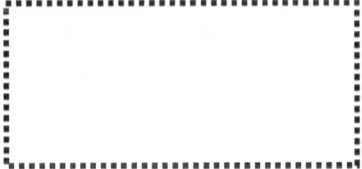

Keep your eyes open for the next 24 hours and try to keep this
count in your head.  Actively keeping watch for things in your
environment keeps your brain active throughout the day!

## BrainChallenge™ - Left Hand Drawing

**Category:** Switch-Up          **Difficulty:** Hard

# Draw your Right Hand with your LEFT HAND

Include rings, wrinkles, cuticles, scars, and anything else you
can see.

## BrainChallenge™ - Right Hand Drawing

Category: Switch-Up        Difficulty: Medium

## Draw your Left Hand with your RIGHT HAND

Try to match the level of detail between the two drawings!

**Category: Creative**     **Difficulty:  Medium**

## Write exactly 25 words about:
## Your Greatest Fear

_____

_____

_____

_____

_____

_____

_____

_____

_____

_____

Expressing yourself within a fixed set of rules can force you to explore different words and sentence structures, which is good brain exercise.

Category: Recall          Difficulty: Easy

# List the LAST NAMES ONLY of six people who you interact with on a daily basis

_____

_____

_____

_____

_____

_____

## Of these people, who is most likely to be harboring an intriguing secret?

_____

Time was, you'd be hard pressed to know a Mister's first name,
but now we are casual enough that it's the last name that
sometimes defies memory.
And it's fun to imagine scandal and adventure

# Name all of the sports teams you've been on

_____

_____

_____

_____

_____

_____

_____

_____

_____

_____

Don't forget intramural, work-related, early school, and
others...  Try to remember details like the uniforms, the
mascots, the coaches...

## BrainChallenge™ - Haiku

| Category: Creative | Difficulty: Medium |
| --- | --- |

## Write a Haiku about Gossip

_____

_____

_____

## Now, write a Haiku about anything, but include the word "Rumor"

_____

_____

_____

### HOW TO HAIKU:

Haiku is a Japanese Poetry Form:
The first line is 5 syllables
The second line is 7 syllables
The third is 5
It need not rhyme!

Writing in verse or haiku forces you to think differently about language, to express yourself in a new way, which is excellent exercise for your brain!

Category: Recall          Difficulty: Hard

## Write in as many languages as you can:
## Excuse Me!

_____

_____

_____

_____

_____

_____

_____

_____

_____

Learning and using languages is great brain exercise.

If you don't know any other languages, why not think of as many ways to say it in your own language?

Category: Recall          Difficulty: Medium

## Draw a Spider

Drawing from Memory pushes you to recall fine detail on familiar objects. How many eyes, how many legs again?

Category:  Switch-Up          Difficulty:  Medium

# Why were the '40s better than the '50s?

_____

_____

_____

_____

_____

_____

_____

_____

_____

_____

Try to make a good case for BOTH SIDES of the argument.  It
forces you to examine your assumptions and bias...

## BrainChallenge™ - Counterpoint

Category: Switch-Up     Difficulty: Medium

## Why were the '50s better than the '40s?

_____

_____

_____

_____

_____

_____

_____

_____

_____

_____

In this case, you may need to overcome strong bias to make
one point over the other. The more you stretch yourself, the
better the exercise for your brain!.

Category: Recall          Difficulty: Medium

## Your mission today:

## Look for birds - how many can you spot?

## (Even in winter, birds abound)

## Bonus Mission:

## Can you name the birds you saw?

_____

_____

_____

_____

_____

Keep your eyes open for the next 24 hours and try to keep this count in your head. Actively keeping watch for things in your environment keeps your brain active throughout the day!

Category: Creative          Difficulty: Easy

## List 7 things that you are NOT.

_____

_____

_____

_____

_____

_____

_____

It can be hard to limit yourself to just 7 things, we know. But try to pick the best!

## BrainChallenge™ - It's a Theory

**Category: Creative**          **Difficulty: Medium**

## Why don't trees grow 1000 feet tall?

_____

_____

_____

_____

_____

_____

_____

_____

_____

The key with "It's a Theory" is to come up with a creative,
possibly plausible, possibly funny explanation to the question
posed. Have fun and use your imagination!

Category: Recall        Difficulty: Medium

## In your BEDROOM:

### How many light switches are there?

_____

### How many light bulbs?

_____

### How many power outlets?

_____

Sometimes the more everyday details of our lives are the
hardest to remember. Give it a try!

## BrainChallenge™ - Twenty Five Words

**Category: Recall**          **Difficulty: Hard**

### Write exactly 25 words about:
### Your Proudest Day

_____

_____

_____

_____

_____

_____

_____

_____

_____

Working creatively within constraints is a great workout.

## BrainChallenge™ Haiku

| | |
|---|---|
| Category: Creative | Difficulty: Easy |

## Write a Haiku about the Earth

_____

_____

_____

## Now, write a Haiku about using the words "River" and "Stones"

_____

_____

_____

### HOW TO HAIKU:

Haiku is a Japanese Poetry Form:
The first line is 5 syllables
The second line is 7 syllables
The third is 5

Writing in verse or haiku forces you to think differently about language, to express yourself in a new way, which is excellent exercise for your brain!

Category: Switch-Up          Difficulty: Hard

## Draw a GIRAFFE with your LEFT HAND

Finally a picture that will really use this tall rectangular
drawing space!

Category: Switch-Up          Difficulty: Medium

## Draw a GIRAFFE with your RIGHT HAND

The two giraffes can be facing eachother if you like.

**Category: Recall**          **Difficulty: Hard**

### Write in as many languages as you can:
### How are you?

_____

_____

_____

_____

_____

_____

_____

_____

_____

Learning and using languages is great brain exercise.

If you don't know any other languages, why not think of as many ways to say it in your own language?

## Why do ghosts prefer to haunt at night?

_____

_____

_____

_____

_____

_____

_____

_____

_____

_____

The key with "It's a Theory" is to come up with a creative, possibly plausible, possibly funny explanation to the question posed. Have fun and use your imagination!

Category: Creative          Difficulty: Medium

## Draw a street sign that indicates:
## "Ferocious Ducks Ahead"

How would you indicate this idea with a simple graphic?

Category:  Recall          Difficulty:  Medium

Hum a Love Song.

(Let it pop into your head!)

Who was the singer?

_____

When was this song popular

_____

Why do you remember THIS SONG?

_____

_____

The melody of a piece of music will stick in your mind far easier than any of the details about the piece, but love songs can bring you back to a point in time. Really try to remember the details about your life at the time.

**Category:  Creative**          **Difficulty:  Easy**

## List 7 things that you hope For

_____

_____

_____

_____

_____

_____

It can be hard to limit yourself to just 7 things, we know.  But
try to pick the best!

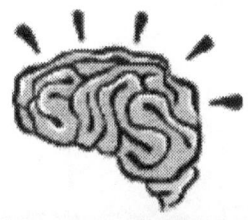

# Congratulations!
## You've completed the
# BrainReady
# BrainChallenge2

Learn the latest brain health & anti-aging
nutritional advice, brain exercises, audio
brain training and much more...FREE at:
www.brainready.com

or send us an email at
info@brainready.com

Thank You!
Jim and Paul

Also Available from BrainReady.com
(printed or download versions):

## BrainFlex Worksheets Volume 1
28 daily brain training worksheets

## BrainChallenge 1
Creative and recall challenges to strengthen
mental acuity the fun and easy way.